WHEELCHAIR
ON THE TRACKS

*My Life With
Cerebral Palsy*

D1456518

WHEELCHAIR ON THE TRACKS

WHEELCHAIR ON THE TRACKS

My Life With Cerebral Palsy

Roger O. Rasmussen

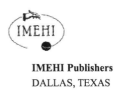

IMEHI Publishers
DALLAS, TEXAS

ACKNOWLEDGMENTS

I would like to thank the following:

The Karcher Staff for getting me started.

United Cerebral Palsy of West Central Wisconsin for their support and encouragement in the production of this book.

Special thanks should be given to Jim Walton for bringing it all together and helping me to realize the final product.

Finally, words alone cannot express the thanks I owe to my family; my mother, Goldie Rasmussen, my sister, Betty Rasmussen Reinke, my brother, Bob Rasmussen, and their families, and to my late father, Richard Rasmussen. Throughout my life they have believed in me, inspired me, and encouraged me. Without them this book would not have been possible.

——Roger O. Rasmussen

Editing and additional rewriting by Jim Walton

Rasmussen, Roger O.
Wheelchair On The Tracks; My Life With Cerebral Palsy/
Roger O. Rasmussen
ISBN13 978-0-9785419-3-4

Printed in the United States of America

TABLE OF CONTENTS

No matter how long we exist, we have our memories. Points in time which time itself cannot erase. Suffering may distort my backward glances, but even to suffering, some memories will yield nothing of their beauty or their splendor. Rather they remain as hard as gems.

——Anne Rice

It is hoped that this book will be of a spiritual nature that will show the love of God I learned as a child

——Roger Rasmussen

Preface
Getting Involved

When we do the best that we can, we never
know what miracle is wrought in our life, or
in the life of another..
———Helen Keller

Everyone struggles for acceptance. Your struggles may be different than mine. They may be physical, or they may be emotional, or psychological. They may be less than mine, or they may be more than mine. To whatever degree you have them, they are real.

Maybe my life and the story of my disabilities — my struggles with not being able to stand or walk, my having to be carried or having to use a wheelchair seem much different than your life. Maybe when you went to school all of your classes were on one floor, and you can't envision having to slide on your butt and bump down the stairs one by one to get to your next class. But, no doubt, you too have faced some difficulties in your life. You know the frustration of not being able, or not being allowed to do or to participate in something you really wanted to do. You know how it feels to be humiliated, to be different, or odd, or hurt. You also have had times when you felt left out, or overlooked.

i

You know what it feels like not to be accepted, not to be part of the "in group". We are all unique and different, but it is difficult for some to appreciate the differences of others. They don't see you as important, or part of the mainstream. Often, others don't know what to do or how to act when they are around you. Maybe they stare, talk softly, or just ignore you. They're afraid of saying the wrong thing, and so they may say nothing at all.

My reason for writing a book is not to condemn anyone. I'm convinced that most people want to do the right thing, but they just don't know what to do when confronted by someone with a severe disability. My hope is that by writing my story it will help you better understand the person who has cerebral palsy, and beyond that, generate an awareness of the needs and challenges that a person who has any disability must face. I believe that early childhood experiences often lead to difficulties later in life.

After reading the story of my life thus far, you may not think it a success story. But no story and no life is either a failure or success until the final chapter is written. At times, my reactions and attitudes have been less than exemplary, and my behaviors less than commendable. I have been locked up in psychiatric wards, and have had to deal with everything involved with institutional confinement. It is not my intention to paint a false picture of my life, or to hide my faults. It is my intention that this book be an honest and open look into my life. I hope by telling my story, as best as I can remember it happened, you will find some examples to follow, and some to avoid.

This is not a book of answers, for I've come to realize that we don't always have the answers. Sometimes all we have are the questions.

I've questioned God – Not "if" there is a God, but I have asked Him, "Why?" "Why did this happen to me?" "Did Roger sin?", "Am I a bad person – am I worse than others?" And I know I am not the only one who questions. I understand someone even wrote a book asking, "Why do bad things happen to good people?" Only if there is another life, a heaven, does it all make sense. If this present physical world is all there is, then there are no answers. No, I cannot be a cynic, I must believe. There IS hope of a better place and a better day!

> *There is nothing so pitiful as a young cynic*
> *because he has gone from knowing nothing*
> *to believing nothing.*
> ——Maya Angelou

In the meantime, we are, each one, who we are, and it is important that we face our individual problems, and challenge our unique circumstances. I cannot change the fact that I have cerebral palsy, and you may not be able to alter the things that limit you. What we can do, is address the lack of services available for those with disabilities. We can work for better laws and better enforcement of laws, such as the Americans with Disabilities Act of 1990 (ADA). And we can become better informed so we can better inform our communities.

Many are not aware that there are over 54 million Americans with physical or mental impairments that significantly limit their daily activities.

I hope the telling of my story will change people's attitudes, give the reader a positive view of people who have a disability, encourage you to vote for candidates that will help the cause of people with disabilities, and inspire everyone to take time to learn more about cerebral palsy. Cerebral palsy is what I have, not who I am. Cerebral palsy does not define me, and your disability should not define you. Become involved. Make your community, your state, and our world a better place for the people with disabilities and everyone else to live.

Have patience with everything unresolved in your heart and try to love the questions themselves as if they were locked rooms or books written in a very foreign language. Don't search for the answers, which could not be given to you now, because you would not be able to live them. And the point is, to live everything. Live the questions now. Perhaps then, someday far in the future, you will gradually, without even noticing it, live your way into the answer.

———Rainer Maria Rilke in *Letters to a Young Poet*

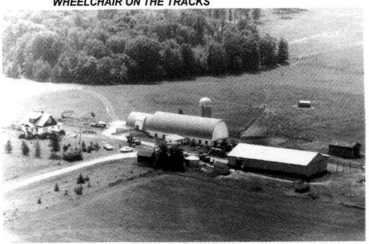

Rasmussen Family Farm

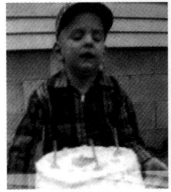

3rd Birthday

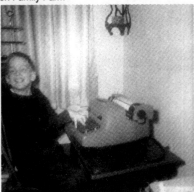

Home school

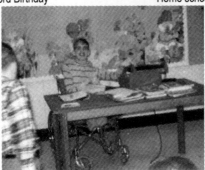

Sunny Skies School

Chapter I
Childhood

*A child's kiss set upon thy sighing lips, shall
    make thee glad;*
*A poor man served by thee, shall make thee
    rich;*
*A sick man helped by thee, shall make thee
    strong;*
*Thou shalt be served thyself by every sense
    of service which thou renderest.*
——Elizabeth Barrett Browning

My earliest recollection of my childhood was hearing aunts, uncles, friends, neighbors, and strangers asking my parents, "Do you think Roger will ever walk?" This was a question my parents and I would hear again and again during the first years of my life.

I grew up on a dairy farm in Baldwin, Wisconsin with my parents, Richard and Goldie Rasmussen, one older brother, Bob, and an older sister, Betty. I was born in 1957 in Baldwin, Wisconsin. My twin brother, Ronnie, died at birth. I was diagnosed with cerebral palsy at the age of one. Around that same time, our farm was hit by a tornado. An enormous amount of destruction and need for rebuilding was left behind by the

1

tornado. As my family struggled to rebuild, I was struggling to learn to crawl and walk.

For most of my childhood, I would go every year for checkups to the University of Wisconsin hospital in Madison. From age two until five, I could walk, but only in parallel bars. Years of wondering and reasoning have brought me to the conclusion, that if you didn't have the ability or the skill to perform a task, you do not miss it. Because the only walking I ever did was as a child—and then only in parallel bars—I do not know what it is like to walk as an able-bodied person. Therefore, How can I miss what I never could do? I can only wonder and imagine what it is like to walk. On the other hand, when later in life, I was told that I could no longer "eat", that, to me, was a big disability and is something I greatly miss.

Family is something else I miss, when it is taken away. In September of 1963, when I was six, I was sent to a special school for handicapped people in Eau Claire, Wisconsin. The school was 40 miles away from my family. I would go down on Monday, live with a foster family during the week, and return home on Friday. I was only able to spend the weekend with my family. I cried day and night because I missed my family. I lasted two weeks, and then the school told me to go home. It was at this time that I got my first wheelchair.

2

Later that fall, my parents and the state worked hard to get me into a regular kindergarten class in the Baldwin-Woodville school district. I was so excited. From the middle of October to Christmas I went to kindergarten in a regular school. Then abruptly I had to leave. I wondered why? All anyone would tell me was that there were people on the school board that wouldn't let me go to school with non-disabled kids. That hurt me. Before this time, I felt the pain and frustration of my disability, but now, for the first time, I felt rejected and discriminated against solely because of my disability.

When I was eight, I went to Easter Seals Camp Wawbeek, near Wisconsin Dells. Camp Wawbeek is a summer camp for children and adults with many disabilities. I remember that when I was three my mom and I had gone to this camp together, but this time, I was alone and I had problems. I cried day and night. I was supposed to stay for two weeks, but I only lasted five days. They called my home and told my parents to come and get me.

I always knew that later in my life I would return to Camp Wawbeek, because mom and dad said that they felt it was important that I have contact with others who were facing similar struggles and challenges due to their disabilities. And so in 1973, when I was 16, they made

3

me go back to Camp Wawbeek.

I remember my anxiety and fear during the weeks leading up to when I would leave for camp. There were tears and bad behaviors, but I found that when I got to camp this time, I enjoyed it. Of course I remember the ice cream, and the water fights that made this trip a little more fun! After that, I continued to go to camp for the next ten years. I think this is where I first learned that I wanted to help and work with people living with a disability.

In the fall of 1965, after a year and a half of trying different foster homes in Eau Claire, a teacher, Mrs. Larson, started visiting my home near Baldwin for an hour a day. I hated it. At the same time, many of my family members; aunts and uncles in an effort to help me learn to adjust to staying away from home, would keep me overnight. Sometimes for days. I fought having to stay away from home. I felt insecure and afraid and at those times.

Looking back, and comparing my high school years with the time when a teacher came to my home for an hour a day and taught me, I wondered why these experiences were so different? I remember hating having to be taught at home and the fact that I was not allowed to study with other kids. High school was better, as I was with other kids. Another big difference, is that at home

4

there seemed to be no motivation to do a good job.

In contrast, life on a dairy farm, provided me with many exciting things to do. I didn't let the fact that I couldn't walk keep me from going to the barn. When my dad went to milk the cows, I would pester him to take me along. I was in the barn a lot. I had my own pig and piglets. I even remember naming one after my aunt.

I went for rides with my father in his truck. Because I couldn't walk, I would sometimes stay in the truck and wait for what seemed like hours for my father to come back. If trials bring about patience, then I think people with disabilities should be some of the most patient people in the world.

I drove tractor and sometimes herded cattle.

I remember that from a very early age I went to a small Baptist church in Hersey, Wisconsin. I learned to trust the Lord. I went to church on Sunday and worked the rest of the week. I think I will never forget the pastors and the teachers who ministered at that little church. I felt accepted in the church. I experienced the truth that in God's sight all believers are brothers and sisters. We were family, and the Hersey church exemplified the love and acceptance that God desires in every church.

Often, the whole church would get together and

have fellowship dinners. In the North, we call them "potluck", in the South, I understand, they call them "covered dish" dinners. It was then that I truly saw the church as a family. Looking back, I don't miss the food, but I miss the people who became like my family—truly they were "my brothers and sisters in the Lord". In my actual family, my mother made sure we all went to church.

I will always remember a Sunday morning after the death of a dear member of the church. As I sat in back, I observed two of the oldest members sitting in front reverently, respectfully, unashamedly remembering their dear departed friend. This is true Christian love.

If I had a main topic for this book it would be, "Don't pity me because I have cerebral palsy, pity more the person whose body is well, but who is not well of spirit."

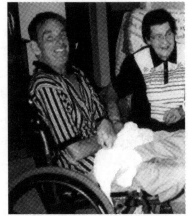

Here I am with my mother

Chapter II
Public School

A true friend knows your weakness but shows you your strengths; feels your fears but fortifies your faith; sees your anxieties but frees your spirit; recognizes your disabilities but emphasizes your possibilities.
——William Arthur Ward

In 1970, it worked out that I could go back to the public elementary school. The school was called, Greenfield Elementary School in Baldwin, Wisconsin. I started out in the Special Education room. I will never forget going out onto the playground for recess on that first day. All the kids stopped playing and stared at me. I had an aide, Mrs. Boldt, who was at my side most of the time, but I felt uneasy, unprotected and all alone. Looking back many, many times it was frustrating, especially as I got older and further along in school. I often thought of college and wondered how I would handle it without the help of my aide.

Within two weeks after the start of school, I was put into a regular class at Greenfield. Back then they didn't call it "mainstreaming". But I fought to stay in the mainstream, and some of the kids I went into class with that day were the same kids I would graduate with years later.

I was at Greenfield from the fall of 1970 to the spring of 1973. I had all the classes the other kids had. The only special therapy I had was speech. Surprising as it may seem, my favorite class was Physical Education. By this time, I had become very close to my aide who started with me in the fourth grade, while I was still in homebound teaching. I took the fourth grade twice; once at home, and again at Greenfield.

Greenfield was a new school with all the rooms on one floor. The teachers were very nice and quite friendly. I remember particularly Mr. Juza and Mrs. Benson. Some of the kids were friendly—some were not. Some made fun of me, but I tried to not let it bother me when they were unkind.

At the end of my sixth grade year, there was a problem. The seventh and eighth grade classes at the school where I was to go were upstairs, and the school administrators didn't think I could attend that school. So I had to go back to a school in Eau Claire. That meant I would have to go to school forty miles from home, and once again be away from my mother and father.

I would travel to Eau Claire on Monday and stay until Friday. It was at this same time that I went back to Camp Wawbeek. Between school and going to camp, I proved something important to myself—I could stay away from home!

In Eau Claire, my soon to be brother-in-law, Dennis, helped me find a home. But it was not long before I found out that the specialized school I was going to did not have the capability to meet my needs. If I was to stay on, I would have to go to yet another junior high in Eau Claire.

It was at this time that I was permitted to return to the Baldwin-Woodville School District. The school I would go to was in Woodville. It was an old school with three stories. I had classes on all three levels and the only way I could go up or down the stairs from class to class was to slide up or down each step on my butt.

You may wonder if this would bother me or be hard on me, but it wasn't. I had been going up and down the steps at home, a two-story farm house with a basement, and at church for a long time. I fit in with the other students very well, and the steps weren't a problem for me. I did try to leave class ahead of the other kids, so I could get to the next class on time.

> *So nigh is grandeur to our dust,*
> *So near is God to man,*
> *When Duty whispers low, Thou must,*
> *The youth replies, I can.*
> —Ralph Waldo Emerson

9

Eighth grade was a memorable year. It is easy for me to remember my first day because it happened to be the same day that we took our family picture in Menomonie. That would be the last family picture of mom, dad, and the three of us kids before the death of my father.

I was happy to be back in school and with the classmates that I had started with at Greenfield. This time, however, was different because I had no aide.

I tried it alone for a month using a typewriter. It didn't go well, and the teachers said that it wouldn't work. So my aide from Greenfield came back. But I was getting older and more independent, and it was hard to get used to having an aide again. I struggled for years with thinking of always having to depend on someone else to help me.

Looking back now, I realize it was a good thing. I don't know how I would have gotten along, or where I would be without the help of this aide. At Greenfield, she did a lot of reading to me, and all of my writing. The teachers at Greenfield didn't like the fact that the aide read to me. This was very frustrating to me as I didn't understand why this would bother them. I usually worked by the library, and spoke my assignments out loud. I didn't like books on tapes.

Because of my cerebral palsy it is hard for me to express or verbalize what I'm thinking. The words were in my mind, but I struggled to speak the words clearly. Some of my teachers from high school would no doubt be surprised if they knew I was writing this book. I ended the eighth grade with my aide still carrying my wheelchair up and down the three-story building. Next year, I was to start high school.

As I look back upon my life, one of my loves is sports, especially high school sports. This may come from the fact that I looked up to my brother, Bob. I was only six when Bob played football in high school. One year, they won the conference championship. I went to all the games, even when it was cold. And believe me it can get very cold in Wisconsin! I remember my mom bundling me up in several pairs of pants, and two coats. I continued to go to both football and basketball games for years, even after Bob had graduated. This was something I enjoyed a lot. To this day, some of my favorite TV watching is the state high school championships from Minnesota and Wisconsin.

One Friday night, Baldwin-Woodville was to play Spring Valley. I wanted to go, but Bob who was now in his first year of college didn't want to take me along. I'm pretty sure Baldwin-Woodville lost the game. They lost all their games that year. That was before Jack

11

Scholz took over. Coach Scholz won three state championships—all after I graduated from high school.

As I entered into my junior high years, I had an idea
about being a manager for the basketball team. I talked
to the basketball coach. He agreed to let me help out
with the practices. My parents wouldn't let me go to the
away games, but I could stay late to help out with the
practices, and I made sure that I went to all the home
games.

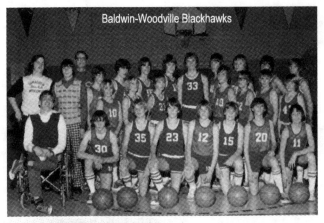

Baldwin-Woodville Blackhawks

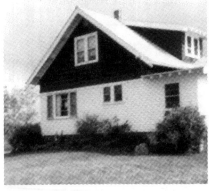

My childhood home

Chapter III
High School

We know not what the path may be as yet by
us untrod;
But we can trust our all to Thee,
Our Father and our God.

——William Josiah Irons

I went into high school in 1975, and did so with great excitement and anticipation. I knew that the possibility of college still lay ahead of me. I would attend a new school in Baldwin where there were not as many stairs, but when I went up and down the steps, it was still on my butt. Mrs. Boldt was also still with me. I read all my assignments myself, and spoke all my sentences out loud so my aide could write them down on paper.

If you have a disability, you only want to be given an opportunity to succeed. You don't want to be given something out of pity. I don't remember what grade it was, but I remember asking one of my teachers, "Did I earn this grade, or did you give it to me because I'm in a wheelchair?" I didn't want to be given a grade that I didn't earn.

I had to work hard on my school work and assignments. Most of my classes were very challenging. I

13

often wonder what my teachers thought of having me in their class, or what they would think if they knew me now. I especially wonder if my English teacher knew I was writing a book, would she laugh, or would she be proud of me? I didn't read many books when I was in school. I recall that, for one English class I managed to get through only reading articles. I had to take a lot of math classes, some more than once. I took Geometry and failed. I also remember taking a Health Careers class.

Even though my aide did my writing, the notes in the classes were taken by other students. Some were good note takers. I remember I paid fifty cents to one student to copy some class notes for me. He said he would collect at the class reunion—he never showed up. I still owe Bill fifty cents, with interest.

School would usually start in early August. We had an outdoor swimming pool, and I remember having great fun pushing a girl named Jill into the pool. Another thing I remember clearly is that I would hold the library door for students and when the principal's daughter would approach, I would quick shut the door. I guess we all played our share of pranks in high school, and I enjoyed a little mischief as much as anyone.

One of the highlights of my senior year, was drama class and the Christmas play, *A Christmas Carol*, by

14

Charles Dickens. We had two performances on a Saturday afternoon in December. I was the Spirit of Christmas Past, and I rolled out in an old wooden wheelchair. This was great fun for me. I felt a part of the cast and of the school. It showed me that given a chance, I could uphold my part and contribute to the whole. I now realize we can all do our part. The more we take part and contribute to our family, to our church, and to our community, the more society and people will begin to understand the needs of people with disabilities. Use your creativity to express yourself and to help others.

The day of the drama performances, I was waiting with the teacher and her friend. The friend was a small boy who was to play Tiny Tim. The teacher was called away, and I was left alone with the boy for about two hours. I had had a rough week with some depression, but I played with the boy hoping to keep him interested. It turned out we had a lot of fun. Several months later, the teacher told the class that that the young boy had an uncle who had recently become a quadriplegic, and the boy had shied away from his uncle. Though the teacher didn't say it directly, she made it sound like because the boy had spent time with me that day, he was more relaxed around his uncle. The uncle was very appreciative.

Physical Education class was my favorite subject.

That may seem strange as pretty much the only thing I did was watch the other kids workout. That meant that I had a lot of time to visit with the teacher, Mr. Scholz. We often stereotype people by their job, the home they come from, the color of their skin, their abilities, or disabilities, or their position in life. I discovered, you can learn a lot more than just sports by talking to a Physical Education teacher.

I hated volleyball, but floor hockey was fun because I got to drop the puck. Life is a lot more interesting and fun when you are a part of the action. My biggest problem turned out to be the locker rooms. They were downstairs, so I always tried to follow the old cliché, "Don't sweat it!", as I wasn't able to shower at school. Occasionally, I would have to go downstairs to the locker room. That meant Mr. Scholz would get a workout as he bumped me down the stairs in my wheelchair.

During Junior High Phy. Ed. in Woodville, we had to walk downtown to the bowling alley. That meant one of the other kids would have to push me in my wheelchair. It turned out that this was a great opportunity for them to pay me back for some of the pranks I had pulled on them. Once, as a joke, they pushed me into a snow bank. Another time, they tied me up to a door knob in the basement locker room. I yelled and yelled for help before the Phy. Ed. teacher finally came to rescue me. I

16

remember being placed under the bleachers in Senior Phy. Ed. class, and the times I played bloody knuckles with the other boys. For the most part it was all in good fun. The pranks didn't seem cruel. They gave me a sense of belonging – of being "one of the guys". And mostly I gave as good as I got. I know that people and the pranks they play, at times can be cruel, but being cruel should never be fun.

While in junior high, I helped the high school basketball team by taping the radio broadcast of the games. Once I got into high school, I would stay after school to watch the football team practice. One time, as I was watching a practice drill from my wheelchair, I got run over by a couple of players. I still wonder if that was an accident, or if they were giving me my payback!

And then, there was the time someone tied my wheelchair to a 4-wheeler. Boy did we fly!! I seldom let barriers get in the way of my having fun.

The month of November was the highlight of my freshman year. This was the month I was in my sister's wedding. She looked so beautiful. I teased her by saying that I could hardly believe it was really her.

November is also the month of Thanksgiving. Dad was still alive at that time, and he came up with the idea of us all going to Michigan to see my brother, Bob. I did have the week off from school and could have used

17

the break as my classes were very difficult. And then, there was the big basketball game against Amery which I wanted to go to. I objected and said I didn't want to miss the game. As it turned out, it didn't do me any good to put up a fuss, we went to Michigan and had a good time. This was the first time I met my brother's fiancée, Sherrie. She and Bob married a year-and-a-half later.

November of my Freshman year, was also the month I became manager of the Baldwin-Woodville basketball team. During my first years as manager, I didn't have a lot of friends. Maybe this was because I wasn't able to go to the away basketball games until my junior and senior years. Before then, my parents didn't want to let me travel to the away games, and even then, the principal objected.

The basketball teams that I managed were so bad that they lost most of their games. On the other hand, the girl's teams were good. I used to sometimes tease them and cheer for the opposing team.

It wasn't until my senior year that I was able to begin going to the movies and such with other kids. I went to my senior prom with a girl—she was just a friend. She said that a lot of people at school looked up to me. At the time, I couldn't understand why. I was really surprised a little later when they gave me a plaque at an

18

high school assembly. They said it was because I had more school spirit than anybody else. As I think back on it now, there was a lot of school pride, and loyalty, and more patriotism at that time. A lot of things are changing. One wonders, what school spirit and loyalty really mean today? Are they as important as they once were?

> *When you're part of a team, you stand up for your teammates. Your loyalty is to them. You protect them through good and bad, because they'd do the same for you.*
> ——*Yogi Berra*

During the summer of my sophomore year, I began career testing in preparation for life after graduation. I had a job evaluation at the University of Wisconsin-Stout in Menomonie. I also had Occupational Therapy and Physiotherapy (OT/PT) evaluation at the University of Minnesota. In the summer of 1978, I worked at a workshop in New Richmond, Wisconsin. At the time, I remember being frustrated and hating just about everything. All I could think about was graduation. My goal upon graduation was to get my own apartment and live on my own. In preparation I even took a personal class on cooking.

In August of 1978, I started my senior year. It was

a difficult year for me. I was confused and depressed. I didn't know what was going to happen in my future. Would I go to college? Would I get a job? Where would I live?

In the spring of 1979, I graduate from Baldwin-Woodville High School. I'm sure some of them thought that moment would never come. When I rolled out onto the stage and got my diploma, everyone stood up and clapped. It was a tremendous thrill to graduate along with my classmates.

I had a big party, but even then I was scared. What was going to happen in my future?

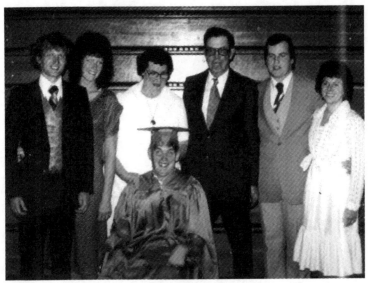

High School Graduation

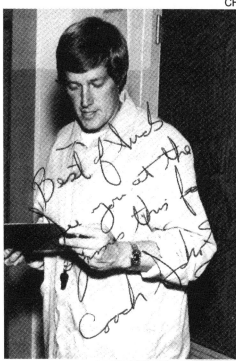

Coach Scholz
Dept. Head—
Physical Education
Boys Phy—Ed.

The Graduate

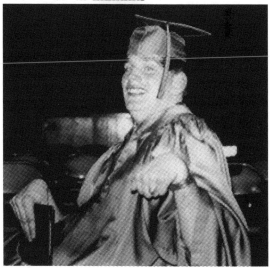

21

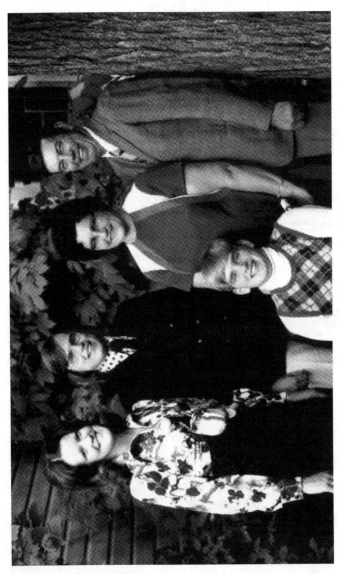

Family picture

Chapter IV
Courage Center

Lord, be Thou near and cheer my lonely way;
With Thy sweet peace my aching bosom fill;
Scatter my cares and fears; my griefs allay,
And be it mine each day
To love and please Thee still.
—Pierre Corneille

In August of 1979, I had a complete evaluation at the University of Wisconsin hospital in Madison. This would prove to be an important evaluation because back then the Standard Aptitude Test (SAT) did not seem to matter, or at least I don't recall hearing a lot about the SAT. They gave me a multitude of tests and sent me to an actual college class for a trial. I took notes using a tape recorder, and later typed them up on a typewriter. The tests and my being able to successfully attend this class proved that I could take college courses. I didn't go to college right away, but the idea of going to college stuck with me for many years. The outcome of it was my going to the Courage Center, a nationally known transitional rehabilitation and resource center for people with disabilities, in Golden Valley, Minnesota.

From April 1980 to April 1981, I attended Courage

23

Center. It was there that I begin to show signs of terrible anger. In my anger, I hurt some people. I had extensive therapy. I became involved in doing some volunteer work out in the community. My interest in basketball continued. I became manager for the Rolling Gophers basketball team.

After a time, I began sensing that other people on the basketball team were making fun of me. This bothered me a lot. I became even more determined that I would make it on my own. I took more therapy. This time, specifically to help me cook for myself. They made me cookware adapted specifically for my use. Meanwhile, I got out into the community at every chance I could.

In January of 1981, I found an apartment in downtown Minneapolis and moved away from the Courage Center. At the time, there were no attendants available, and so I moved into the apartment by myself. I kept in contact with the Courage Center and was finally able to find an attendant.

I did all my own grocery shopping. I attended a Baptist church and found some good companions. But after only a month, I realized that I was having trouble managing my money. I was scared as I didn't want to have to go back to the Courage Center. When I was at the Courage Center, and before moving into the apartment, the center threatened many times that I would have to be put into a nursing home. I did not want to go to a nursing home. It scared me to think about it.

One day when I was still in the apartment, I accidentally hit the water pipes in the bathroom and water sprayed everywhere. I had to move back to the Courage Center and give up my apartment. I felt as if I had failed.

After the failure of apartment living, the people at the Courage Center seemed all the more determined to send me to a nursing home. Someone asked me what it is like to live in a nursing home. For the person who has a disability, but who is not old, it is extremely hard to be placed into a nursing home. Nursing homes are designed to care for the elderly. A young person with a disability needs rehabilitation and help to transition to a more meaningful and productive life.

In the spring of 1981, for the first time, I was locked up in a psychiatric ward in Minneapolis. I was sent there for getting mad and striking out at people at the Courage Center. There would follow many such incidents in my life.

I struck out at people, because I did not want to go to the nursing home. All I could think of was that I wanted to go back to Wisconsin and live with my mom and dad. I was locked up for about a week. During this time, I got lots of encouragement from my family and was able to return to the Courage Center.

About a month later, after a time of being depressed and trying to put my life back together, I fainted on the floor of the Center. Scared of what they would do to me, I called up the pastor of my small country church. I asked him to take me away from there and drive me to my parents farm. He agreed. I fainted again in the car.

That night I talked with my parents about my situation and my fears. I wanted to stay with them, but they knew it wouldn't work. It must have broken their hearts to tell me that they couldn't take me back. I felt that they didn't want me back.

I tried committing suicide by slashing my wrists with a kitchen knife. When that failed, I agreed to go to a psychiatric ward as long as it was not in Minnesota. I was admitted to the psychiatric ward at Sacred Heart Hospital in Eau Claire, Wisconsin. I still wasn't happy, and I hit out and exhibited a great deal of bad behavior. Finally, I was given two options: I could go to another long-term psychiatric ward, or I could go to Maple Manor nursing home in New Richmond, Wisconsin.

Chapter V
Maple Manor

Though to-day may not fulfill
All thy hopes, have patience still;
For perchance to-morrow's sun
Sees thy happier days begun.
——Paul Gerhardt

In May of 1981, I arrived at Maple Manor nursing home. It was about a sixty-bed facility filled mostly with elderly people, with a friendly staff. What I liked most, was that it was only half-an-hour from Baldwin where I went to high school, and it wasn't far from my family. After about a week, I started to wheel uptown by myself in my wheelchair on a regular basis. I bought things like the paper and junk food. I also began psychiatric therapy from the St. Croix County mental health facility. They helped me look back at what went wrong at the Courage Center.

Realizing a need to resolve some of the issues and things that had gone wrong while at Courage Center, I got in contact with the Center. I received an apology from the Center, and was able to get to the bottom and lay to rest some of the issues that had been troubling me.

27

While in the hospital, in Eau Claire, I got in contact with United Cerebral Palsy of West Central Wisconsin. They were a great help to me.

In the summer of 1981, I began working on a volunteer basis at the Wisconsin Indianhead Technical Institute (WITI). I had contacted them six months before I went to the Courage Center. In the fall of 1981, I tried taking classes at the Wisconsin Indianhead Technical Institute (WITI). The classes I took were English, Sociology, The American Constitution, and some computer classes. For the most part, I would take a taxi to class, it cost me $3.00 a trip.

I returned to New Richmond and one of the first things I did was to start to go to football, basketball, and baseball games. I was so into high school sports that I even went to the practices and sat in on the team meetings. You may wonder why I went to the high school games and hung around the kids in New Richmond, and, later, throughout my years in Baldwin. It was to show the kids that I supported them. I think it is important for everyone to show our youth that we are interested in and support them and their activities.

I did not want to sit around and do nothing. This is a part of who I am. It is how I want to live. The baseball games were especially fun, because New Richmond is a baseball town. I have a disability, but I want to be

28

involved and a part of the community.

I went to meetings about local area referendums. I got involved in the local theater group. I also became involved in the local cable TV committee. At the time, New Richmond didn't have cable TV. We began investigating the possibility of bringing cable TV to New Richmond. I must admit that my motives may not have been entirely altruistic. After all, cable would bring the Green Bay Packers' football games to New Richmond's TV sets. It didn't happen quickly, but the town was ultimately successful in getting cable, even though I had left and was not there to see it. We don't always see the results of our efforts, but I am sure of one thing, it is never wrong to try. Sometimes we may never know what good may result from our trying.

During my time in New Richmond, I met a friend, Jack Boor. He was a principal of New Richmond High School. I think he is now retired. If this book does one thing, I hope to finds friends like Jack. Life is short, and we lose touch with our friends much too soon.

In the spring of 1982, I started working on an accounting degree through Wisconsin Indianhead Technical Institute. It was to be a two-year self-paced degree. At the time, I didn't own a computer and did all my work on a typewriter. What would take an able-bodied student one semester, would take me a year. Because I

was involved with the Wisconsin Department of Rehabilitation, they paid my tuition and transportation.

Maple Manor was a friendly nursing home and I had
a lot of fun there. I stayed for two years, but I wasn't
fully happy, and I still thought I could live in my own
apartment.

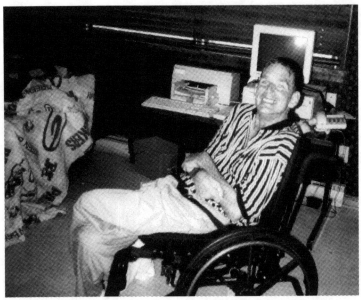

Notice the Green Bay Packers blanket—**Go Packers!**

Chapter VI
A Hard Time

Character cannot be developed in ease and quiet. Only through experience of trial and suffering can the soul be strengthened, ambition inspired, and success achieved.
———Helen Keller

As I said in the last chapter, I was still determined to live in my own apartment. It hadn't worked out well when I tried it before, but I thought my first apartment was just a mistake. I began looking in the paper for an apartment. I could not afford most of the apartments, , and the rest were unavailable. I looked until February of 1983 before I found one in New Richmond and signed the lease. I interviewed a number of aides and picked a couple I thought would be suitable.

Soon, I discovered that I was not left to be completely on my own. My adventure had become kind of a community effort. The high school got me a ramp for my wheelchair. My mom and dad moved some of my stuff into the apartment. It seemed everybody helped, and before I knew it, everything was in place and in order.

My aides had not arrived yet, but I was so excited,

31

that I moved in anyway. I stayed there alone for a couple of days and one night. Then, I began feeling anxious and went back to sleep at Maple Manor. The next day, I felt depressed, and I cried a lot. That night, I went back to my parents' house.

The next morning, I woke up depressed. I began acting badly, cried a lot, and hit out at my parents. I said I didn't want my apartment. They called the doctor and finally got something to calm me down. Up to this point, I had taken no medication for my anger or depression. For a day and a half I continued to strike out at my parents. I went back to Maple Manor, and at first, I didn't strike out.

After the failure at living in the apartment in New Richmond, I was depressed for three weeks straight. I began to act out at Maple Manor and had to leave. I was locked up in the St. Croix Healthcare Center with some severely mentally disturbed people. I could not return to Indianhead Technical Institute where I was studying accounting.

I was confused and I started misbehaving at the healthcare center. I knew I couldn't go back to Maple Manor. In desperation I ran away from the St. Croix Healthcare Center with the help of a taxi. I went to my parents' house. This didn't last a week. I ended up at Sacred Heart Hospital again. The next day, they transferred me to the Dunn County Healthcare Center. I was locked up there for three months. I would hit people and misbehave. They put me in restraints in a room that had pink walls, and kept me in the room overnight.

They eventually committed me to a hospital in Owen, Wisconsin. I was there for six months. My parents would come to see me on Sundays. Owen was a good place for me as there were a lot of young people. When I acted out, they put me in restraints, took me out of my wheelchair, and put me at the end of a long hall. Once again, my cerebral palsy had separated me from others. Lacking companionship and reaching back, I kept in contact with some of my friends in New Richmond.

> *The chief pang of most trials is not so much the actual suffering itself, as our own spirit of resistance to it.*
> ——Jean Nicolas Grou

Over the six months I was at Owen, I got better and stopped hitting and acting out. I learned how to weave on a loom. I bought a radio that had a TV on it and listened to the football games. I also got a job working in a cafeteria washing chairs. In those six months, it was the first time in many months that I wasn't on any medications. I began looking back to see what I had done

33

and tried to figure out what it was that I really wanted out of life.

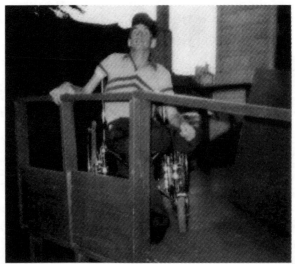

Ramp

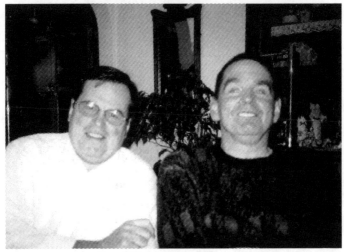

With my brother, Bob.

Chapter VII
Return to Baldwin

Keep your eyes on the stars
and your feet on the ground.
——Theodore Roosevelt

After the six months at Owen, I moved back home with my parents to wait for an opening at the Baldwin Nursing Home. In the spring of 1984, I found an old hotel in Baldwin which had a lot of elderly people living there. I got a room and lived there from 1984-1992.

It was about this time that I found out I was going to be an uncle for the first time. That was great news, and it came at an especially exciting time in my life. It was also a time when I had many things on my mind. I was back "home", in Baldwin, and spending all my time getting reacquainted with former teachers and old friends. I got to know Baldwin all over again. I spent much time in those years at the Dairy Queen and at the Super Valu store eating junk food. I was busy twenty-four seven trying to catch up and put my life back in order. I built a ramp from materials that I had left over from the New Richmond apartment. I attended a mental health treatment group two times a week, for about a year. Then, in the fall of 1984, my Grandmother died.

35

But life went on. I started working at St. Croix Industries; a workshop for people who have a disability. We sorted various things and did a lot of different jobs. I learned a lot at St. Croix Industries. I had worked there the summer of my junior year in high school and didn't like it. But when I went back in 1985, my outlook had changed, and I liked it.

Three years after the death of my father, I was still living in the old hotel in Baldwin. It was located on main street. I had easy access to downtown, and of course, I continued to spend a lot of time going to high school activities like, football, basketball, and baseball. I roamed the streets of Baldwin in my wheelchair (it wasn't electric). It was "Roger powered". I did it with my legs.

One of my biggest problems while living in the old hotel, was transportation. This is a major problem for many who have a disability. At the time, I was working 20 miles away in New Richmond. I got some help with transportation from the Office on Aging, and later I received money from the State to pay drivers to take me to work. This, like so many government sponsored programs, was a complicated process. I often wonder if the desire to reduce all rules, regulations and paperwork to a minimum, and make things simple is really irrational, or if it is the bureaucratic maze that is nonsensical.

I was able to do many things for myself, and even take my own baths. The hotel staff would do my laundry and cook my meals. The staff were very kind to me. One thing I specially remember are the big glasses of milk they gave me.

I got to go to away sports games by the kindness of a man that ran the local newspaper, Tom Hawley. I went to high school with his sister, Mary Hawley. I once promised Mary that if I ever wrote a book, I would mention her name. Promise kept.

And here's a secret, about clothes. The way to get new clothes is to have a sister. Once, my sister, Betty, confiscated an old blue shirt (my favorite) that I wore every time I saw her. We now exchange the shirt, as a joke, for Birthdays and holidays! She still gives me clothes, and she also gives me advice, understanding, encouragement, hope, and hugs!

I stayed at the old hotel for seven years. As time went on, many people moved out and the majority of those who remained at the hotel were people with mental illness. Because I was physically disabled, but mentally competent, I didn't belong. At times, those of us who lived there would have arguments. I recall one time that police had to be called to restore order. They ended up taking one person away.

In my adult life, I have had a lot of problems with

my teeth. You may be thinking, "That doesn't seem like such a big deal, many people have a lot of problems with their teeth." But what are common activities for most, and things the vast majority of people take for granted—such as walking, talking, sitting still, standing up, eating, drinking, swallowing, getting dressed, brushing your teeth, or just going to the dentist—can be an excruciating struggle for a person with cerebral palsy. If achieved, it is only by immense effort. It is almost equally as difficult for the dentist who must examine, clean, x-ray, fill, drill, suction, cap, or crown. Not to mention, do a root canal! I had to go to a special dentist in Eau Claire. Several times I had to be put to sleep so that they could work on my teeth.

After my father died, my family had an auction and sold all of dad's machinery. My mom moved into Baldwin to a house that was also on Main Street, but on the other side of town. I was happy that mom would be moving closer to me, and I thought that Baldwin would be better off with two Rasmussens on Main Street.

In the fall of 1987, I decided to fly out to my brother Bob's in Michigan for Thanksgiving. Flying was much quicker and different than my previous bus trip, with my parents, to Washington DC. We had a great meal at Bob's of turkey and all the trimmings. The next morning, I was taking a shower and accidentally hit the glass

38

shower screen. The door shattered into a million pieces. I had to go to the emergency room for stitches and observation. The rest of the trip was without incident.

Back in Wisconsin, with my work at Stepping Stones I got interested in computers. I often worked on a computer in the office of a man who volunteered with Stepping Stones. I learned a lot of skills there.

I was a very active person. Living and working in both Baldwin and New Richmond. I continued to maintained an avid interest in sports. I became well known all over New Richmond as a dedicated sports fan. An interesting experience happened one day while I was in New Richmond doing work for Stepping Stones, a man drove up, stopped, and asked me about the New Richmond Basketball team. "Do you think they will win or lose?" I had to say that I didn't know.

I tell you this, because both in Baldwin and in New Richmond I was involved in the community. By becoming involved, I got to know people, and they got to know me. I believe everyone, especially those with a disability, need to be involved in their community, so others get to know us as people.

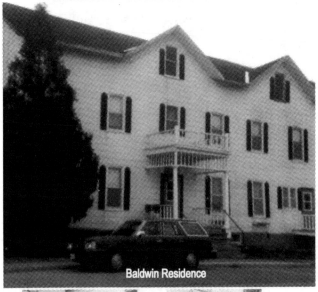

Baldwin Residence

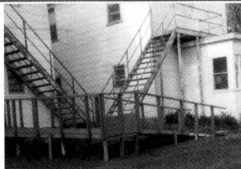

A ramp made the
residence accessible

Riding in town
parade

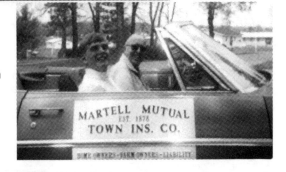

MARTELL MUTUAL
EST 1878
TOWN INS. CO.

40

Chapter VIII
My Favorite Pastimes

*And when it rains on your parade, look up
rather than down. Without the rain, there
would be no rainbow.*

——Jerry Chin

When I lived in the old hotel, and for many years after
that, some of my favorite pastimes were going to the
county fairs and to other community events. If I was
well known in New Richmond, I was very well known
in Baldwin. Baldwin, at that time, had an annual celebration they called, "Dutch Days".

There was a parade, and before the parade there
was the traditional Dutch custom of washing the streets.
The men would take buckets of water and pour the water onto the street. The women would follow sweeping
the streets with brooms. I would help the men pour the
water onto the streets, and at times accidentally throw a
bucket of water onto a person. These "accidents" would
happen quite often. As a matter of fact, to this day, I
still owe a businessman a pail of water — I'm sure he
knows who he is. This is fair warning. "See you at
Dutch Days!"

After the street washing, people in traditional

41

Dutch costumes—complete with wooden shoes—would come dancing down the street. I would ride along and carry spare shoes for the dancers.

There was a park across from the hotel with a gazebo in it. During town celebrations, the park was filled with many people and dozens of food stands. I tried to visit all of them.

During Dutch Days, there were many other activities in town. It seemed every house in town had a garage sale, and I attended every one of them. I would take off the night before the sale, in my wheelchair, and try to get the best bargains before the early birds arrived the next morning. Sometimes it worked, and sometimes it didn't.

Another celebration I enjoyed was Woodville's Norwegian Independence Day Celebration. I rode in the parade on two separate occasions. There was always tons of food. As I got older, I found I could no longer eat like I did when I was younger. Eventually, as you will read later in this book, in chapter 17, I could no longer swallow. I now "eat" by a feeding tube. Now, I have only my memories of mom's cooking, the potluck dinners at the Hersey church, and Woodville's Norwegian Independence Day Celebrations.

In 1994, something happened that I really enjoyed. I attended the WIAA Division Four State Championship football game. The Baldwin-Woodville "Blackhawks"

emerged as the WIAA Division Four State Runner-Up.
As I recall, Baldwin-Woodville going to the State
championships seemed to happen quite often. In 1981,
they were the WIAA Division Three State Runner-Up;
in 1983, the WIAA Quarter-Final Champions; in 1987,
they beat Beloit Turner to become WIAA Division Four
State Champions; in 1988 they were the WIAA Sec-
tional Runner-Up; and in 1992 the WIAA Division Four
State Champions. I was able to get to all the state
championship games. I even traveled to Madison to see
one of the games with a guy who in later years accom-
panied me
on a trip to
Florida.

Baldwin-Woodville Championships
WIAA State Championships
1987 WIAA Division Four State Champions
November 14, 1987: B-W 16, Beloit Turner 8
1992 WIAA Division Four State Champions
November 12, 1992: B-W 11, Mayville 7
WIAA State Appearances
(other than titles)
1981 WIAA Division Three State Runner-Up
1983 WIAA Quarter-Final Champions
1988 WIAA Sectional Runner-Up
1994 WIAA Division Four State Runner-Up
1995 WIAA Level Two Qualifier
1996 WIAA Level One Qualifier
1997 WIAA Level One Qualifier
1998 WIAA Level Two Qualifier
1999 WIAA Level One Qualifier
2000 WIAA Level One Qualifier
2002 WIAA Level Two Qualifier
Middle Border Conference Champions
1963
1970, 1974
1981, 1982, 1983, 1987, 1988
1992
2000
Northwest Football League - Blue Division Champions
1994, 1995

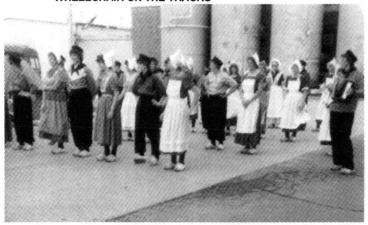

Baldwin, Wisconsin's "Dutch Days"

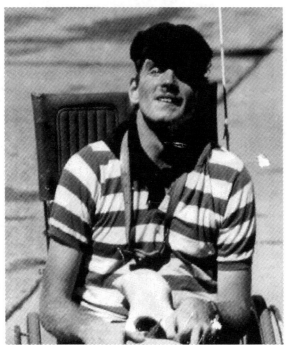

Here I am with a spare wooden shoe for dancers.

44

Chapter IX
Family

The happiest moments of my life have been
the few which I have passed at home in the
bosom of my family.
——Thomas Jefferson

Family is one of God's greatest gifts. My family has always been there for me. Without the love and support of family where would any of us be? They are there when we need help, comfort, or an arm to lean on. Who else is there to share the joys and the milestones in our lives, and yes, to share the sorrows and pain of our bad times? We depend on them when we have a need. If we get mad at them—though they may not say it—they love us anyway. I love my family and am so happy for my brother, Bob, and sister, Betty. Among the most exciting times in my life were the times I found out that their families were expanding, and I was going to be an uncle.

First, it was my brother, Bob, and his wife, Sherrie. They informed our family that they were adopting two boys. At about the same time, my sister, Betty, announced the birth of a boy into their family.

I will never forget a Saturday in 1985 when mom

and dad, "Grandma and Grandpa Rasmussen", were
showing off their two adopted grandchildren, Greg and
Steve, to all the aunts and uncles. At the same time, my
sister, Betty, was showing off her big belly— which
would turn out to be my nephew, Kyle. It felt so good
to be an uncle. It was an exciting day for everyone in
my family.

My mother and my sister are so much alike. Their
love of God and their love for their children is so evi-
dent. They are always giving and sharing their love and
talents by baking cookies for their children, or having
parties for them and their friends.

I don't talk near enough about my mom and my dad
in this book. Richard and Goldie Rasmussen have to be
the finest people, and the best parents anyone could
wish for. The name Rasmussen, was quite well-known
in St. Croix County in the 1960's. I remember my
mother and father's twenty-fifth wedding anniversary.
It was a surprise affair with many church people and
relatives in attendance. Fifteen years later, I was privi-
leged to be at their 40th wedding anniversary.

Being raised on a farm, I herded cows with my
mother, raised pigs, and went to the barn with my father.
It seems my mom is just always there for me, and always has been. Many times there was no one else, but
mom was always there. I sometimes think that when I

was angry and hit out, she was the person I hurt most often. She was always the nearest and closest. Mom is strong of character, godly, hard-working, and wise. I love her a lot. I'm sure there are other great moms— mine is special!

I miss my father a lot. One day I called my parents home. My mom wasn't there. Dad answered the phone and I asked him how he was. He said he had gone to Iowa and bought a pony for the grandkids. He named the pony, "Jude". Bob's family returned that summer and the boys got to ride Jude. Kyle, who was born May 14, 1985, would not know the love of his grandpa, Richard, or enjoy the pony, as dad died September 1986, before Kyle was a year and a half old.

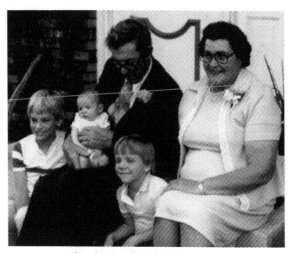

Grandpa and Grandma Rasmussen
With Grandsons:Greg, Kyle and Steve.

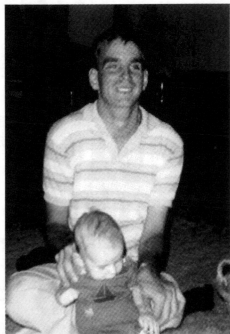

Here I am with
my nephew, Kyle.

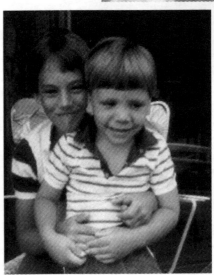

My nephews,
Greg and Steve.

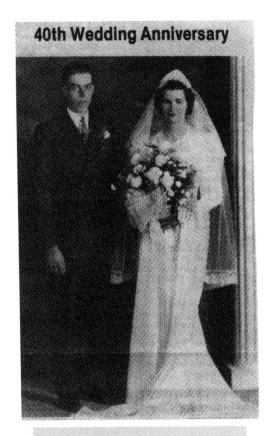

40th Wedding Anniversary

A reception was held for Mr. and Mrs. Richard Rasmussen on Sunday, August 16, 1961 at the Coachman Supper Club in Baldwin, Wisconsin, in honor of their 40th wedding anniversary.

The event was hosted by their children, Robert and Sherrie Rasmussen, Pontiac, Michigan; Dennis and Betty Reinke, Eau Claire, Wisconsin; and Roger Rasmussen, New Richmond, Wisconsin.

49

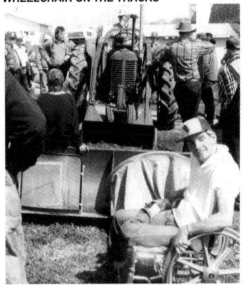

Rasmussen Auction

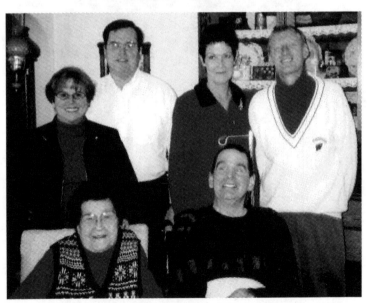

Bob and Betty with their spouses, and my mom and me.

Chapter X
Stepping Stones

We shall not fail or falter; we shall not weaken or tire...Give us the tools and we will finish the job..
—Sir Winston Churchill

They said it was a milestone. I knew there would be many milestones and many opportunities for me to become involved with groups, organizations, and government programs to help people who have a disability or obstacle to overcome in their lives.

While still in high school, in the fall of 1976, I started to work with United Cerebral Palsy. United Cerebral Palsy of West Central Wisconsin was there in my good and bad times. They helped me in every part of my life from finances to emotional support. I was given a counselor, Ruth G., who served as both therapist and advisor. I worked with her till August of 2004. I served on the board of directors, and was also on some of the United Cerebral Palsy telethons.

In 1984, I was to be introduced to an advocate field coordinator, Donna F. It was then, that we started a group called, "Stepping Stones of St. Croix County". Stepping Stones was a group of people with disabilities

51

who worked in the same workshop. We sponsored events such as pancake suppers, and held meetings with decision makers.

Transportation is a major problem for people with disabilities, especially when living in a small town. The range of services offered by small towns is often different from what is offered by larger cities. It is essential that people with disabilities have equal opportunity to participate in the services and programs the town or city offers. We conducted a transportation survey, and found that access for those with disabilities to public transportation to be a major barrier to them becoming contributing members of the community. We had meetings with town officials and other agencies to talk about the problem. They listened, but nothing would come of this for many years. Lesson learned: Not everything happens quickly—be patient, but be persistent.

> *Never give in—never, never, never, never, in nothing great or small, large or petty, never give in except to conviction of honour and good sense. Never yield to force; never yield...*
> ——Sir Winston Churchill

From 1986 to 1989, I worked in the New Richmond office for Stepping Stones. We had a bumper sticker campaign in cooperation with a soft drink company to make others aware of people with a disability. We put on benefit meals to raise awareness and increase funding to meet the needs of the people with disabilities. If there is one thing I would like the readers of this book to take away, it is the importance of doing awareness programs in your community.

There are many ways we can make people aware of the needs of people with disabilities. For example, we went to county fairs to distribute materials regarding people with disabilities. One year, we had a float that was entered in local parades. Every two years, we would drive three hours to Madison, with 30 to 40 people in vans and cars, to take part in a state-wide rally.

One of my favorite things, while working at Stepping Stones, was to put together teen dances. I would hire a DJ and the money raised would go to the Stepping Stones' programs to help those with disabilities.

As our group grew, the advocate coordinator and I returned to my old middle school and did an awareness campaign. No doubt, some of my mischievous ways came back to the mind of my teachers. Thankfully a mischievous past doesn't have to keep us from doing good things today.

The awareness campaign lasted a week. We

53

teamed up with two parents of children with disabilities who used puppets to get the message across. We would go to different towns to find out how accessible each of their buildings were to people with disabilities. We presented plaques to those who had the most accessible buildings. This program was funded for six counties, so we would often meet together with those from other counties for training. We had camping trips and dances. The possibilities are unlimited.

To my thinking, the biggest thing we did (I wish it was done more often today), was to go into the local schools and have awareness month. We would work together with the teachers. The students were divided into several levels which did different things to help them become aware of people with disabilities, and show them how they can relate to someone with a disability. Roughly speaking, the K-3rd grade kids might draw pictures of people with a disability doing things. As a reward they would get grab bags from the local businesses; 4th to 7th grades might make something that a person with a disability could use, and also get a reward for their effort; 8th grade to seniors can write an essay about a person with a disability.

I feel so much of what we learned in Stepping Stones would be an enormous help to individuals with disabilities, and to the schools, companies, communities, and committees who must work together. I hope that through this book, and in person, I am able to pass on the knowledge of what I learned in Stepping Stones.

Stepping Stones held candidate forums where they invited candidates running for elected office to speak on disability issues. As a result, I met a former friend. At one of these forums a man came up to me and said, "Haven't I seen you before?" I thought he must be someone from college. He turned out to be my old boy scout leader from Eau Claire, Joe Plouff. This program also resulted in my being appointed by the governor to the Wisconsin Council of Developmental Disabilities.

The Council made contracts with groups to provide services for the people with disabilities, and also advised the legislature on legislation pertaining to people with disabilities. We developed a three-year plan for our work. As a member of the board, I flew to Madison for meetings.

The government was also going through a rough time, so sometimes I had to fly back on the 8 a.m. Sunday morning flight because it was cheaper. I made these trips by myself. One time when I came back, I was to go to a family reunion. I decided to play a joke on one of my aunts. I put my dirty clothes in a box and gave it to her to wash. She must have caught on to the joke, as she never did wash the clothes.

In 1988, I was appointed and served several years on the Governor's Committee for People with Disabilities. We advised the governor on issues pertaining to people with disabilities, started a camp to teach youth with disabilities, how to influence lawmakers and bring about legislation. We also worked with the Department of Vocational Rehabilitation (DVR). We had representatives for other councils and did a lot of work, including bettering handicap parking. It was a very dedicated and fun group to work with. I would love to someday see them all again: Tom Fell, Wayne Corey, Joe Mosgular, and many others.

It was at this time that the Americans With Disabilities Act of 1990 (ADA) was being enacted. I hope everyone reading this book will become acquainted with this law that requires State and local governments, as well as other non-Federal government agencies to operate their programs so that their services are readily accessible to and usable by people with disabilities.

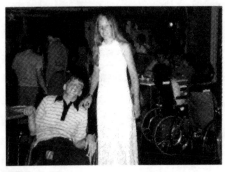

Here I am with a friend from Stepping Stones.

CERTIFICATE OF APPRECIATION

For outstanding service to the

Wisconsin Council on Developmental Disabilities

awarded to

ROGER RASMUSSEN

WCDD Member - 1986-87
Member, Education/Information Committee
and Transportation Task Force

presented on _____ December 10, 1987 _____

Al Salmayer
Chairperson

signature
Executive Director

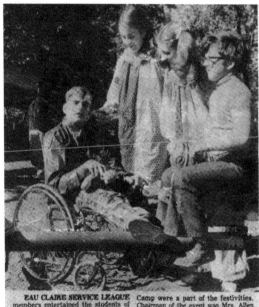

EAU CLAIRE SERVICE LEAGUE members entertained the students of Putnam Heights Achievement Center at Carson Park recently for their annual picnic. Clowns greeted the students, and a visit to the Paul Bunyon Camp were a part of the festivities. Chairman of the event was Mrs. Allen Vann, co-chairman, Mrs. Robert Risberg. Pictured from left Roger Rasmussen, Dorothy Atkinson, Carol Anderson and Jerry Tellstrom.

57

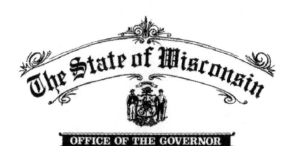

The State of Wisconsin

OFFICE OF THE GOVERNOR

KNOW YE, that I, ANTHONY S. EARL, Governor of the State of Wisconsin, reposing special trust and confidence in his integrity and ability do hereby appoint **Roger Rasmussen** of Baldwin to the **Wisconsin Council on Developmental Disabilities** for a term to expire July 1, 1987.

AND, I hereby authorize the exercise of the powers and the duties of that office according to his discretion.

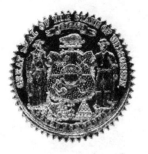

IN TESTIMONY WHEREOF, I have hereunto set my hand and caused the Great Seal of the State of Wisconsin to be affixed. Done at the Capitol in the City of Madison this day, July 15th, in the year of Our Lord, one thousand nine hundred eighty-six.

ANTHONY S. EARL

SECRETARY OF STATE

CHAPTER XI
Dreams Fulfilled

I have a dream that one day every valley shall be exalted, and every hill and mountain shall be made low, the rough places will be made plain and the crooked places will be made straight and the glory of the Lord shall be revealed and all flesh shall see it together.

——Martin Luther King, Jr. –from speech delivered at
the Lincoln Memorial on August 28, 1963

In the fall of 1991, the old hotel begin to fill up with people with more serious mental disabilities. The staff began to yell at the residents more. Looking at my life, I saw that I was living with all old people, or people with mental disabilities. I wanted more for my life. I decided it was time to get my own apartment. I told my county social worker, whom I had become very close to, that I wanted to move into my own apartment. She contacted a local provider of housing for people with disabilities. We started searching for a new apartment for me. This took some time. During this time my behavior was somewhat unstable. I would scream and hit the staff at the hotel, and I ran to my mother's house a lot. Finally, in the summer of 1992, I had to leave the hotel.

59

I decided to go to live with my mother. We had to build a ramp for my wheelchair. I was only to live with my mother for three months.

In the fall of 1992, I moved into my first Baldwin apartment. I had an attendant who would go shopping with me, and we would go for rides and walks together. This attendant would last only three months. My next attendant lasted two years. In spite of that, I learned a lot from him. I would do my own laundry and get my own breakfast. The attendant would fix my supper.

I began working at St. Croix Industries in the summer of 1992. I also started training for a paper shredding job for the county human service office. It was close to the workshop. I started shredding paper for money during the winter of 1993. In the three years that I worked shredding paper for St. Croix County Human Services, I also worked part-time —three days a week— at St Croix Industries.

In the fall of 1993, with the help of an attendant, I started auditing classes at the University of Wisconsin-Stout, in Menomonie, Wisconsin. My first class was a class on World War II. I did very well in the class and enjoyed it. I audited another class and did very well in that class also. It was about this time that I became very interested in the Internet and spent a lot of time on campus searching the internet. My aide was also interested in flying, which may have led to my first, <u>and only</u>, sky-diving experience.

I did a lot of experimenting with a lot of different classes; from desk top publishing to computer classes; I was getting financial aid and so was able to start a degree in psychology. I took many classes and did a lot of typing. Something, today, I don't know that I would be able to do. I even took a class in creative writing, which I think is helping me a lot in writing this book. I loved to do a lot of the psychological experiments. I even took a yoga class.

In the beginning, I ate my suppers on campus, which I enjoyed. I went to the University of Wisconsin-Stout for seven years.

I am forever indebted to the person that influenced me to go to college. If this book encourages one other person with a disability to go on to college, my efforts will have been worth it.

Roger Rasmussen's dream fulfilled

For Roger Rasmussen of 1762 Sixth Avenue, a dream has come true. On September 17th, Roger moved into a new duplex, that was designed specifically with him in mind. Roger has cerebral palsy and uses a wheelchair.

Roger's wheelchair is a familiar sight on the streets of Baldwin. He has lived in the Baldwin area for most of his thirty-some years.

Born and raised on a farm in Wilson, Roger was sent to an Eau Claire special school for a couple of years, but being away from home at the tender age of six and seven was too much for both Roger and his family. He was returned to the B-W school district where a full-time aide helped him complete his education.

"Mrs. Boldt (the aide) was a very important person in my life," Roger says. "She moved with me through every grade until I graduated."

Roger, still an avid fan of the Baldwin-Woodville Blackhawks, was the manager of the basketball team all four years of high school.

When Roger decided to move out of the Baldwin Residence where he had lived for several years, Aurora Residential Alternatives of Menomonie began the search for a home that could be made accessible. When it became clear that nothing was available in Baldwin, it was

Continued from Page 1A

decided to begin construction of the 3 bedroom duplex. Roger was able to live with his mother, Goldie Rasmussen in Baldwin in the meantime.

Planning the move to his new home was a team effort, with staff from Human Services, Aurora and United Cerebral Palsy of West Central Wisconsin meeting with Roger. UCP serves a ten county area which includes Baldwin/Woodville.

Roger has worked with United Cerebral Palsy for 15 years, serving on its Board of Directors for four years.

"UCP has been a great support to

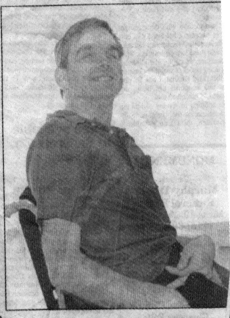

Roger Rasmussen is pictured at his kitchen table in his new home in Baldwin.

CHAPTER XII
LIVING ALONE

*All who call on God in true faith, earnestly
from the heart, will certainly be heard, and
will receive what they have asked and de-
sired, although not in the hour or in the
measure, or the very thing which they ask;
yet they will obtain something greater and
more glorious than they had dared to ask.*
——Martin Luther

In the fall of 1994, the service that provided my aid decided I could live on my own, so my life changed
greatly. I would wake up at five thirty a.m. and work on
the laundry, do my home work, make my own breakfast,
bathe and get ready for work. I was totally on my own
and enjoyed it very much.

I lived by myself for almost a year. After a year of
enjoying an apartment by myself and just having people
come in to help me from time to time, I got a roommate.
I believe this experience taught me an important lesson;
people need to be active and not sit around home a lot.

My new roommate was very different from me. He
wanted to stay in his room all the time. I became aware
of this even before he came to live with me. I heard that

63

he would often misbehave badly when people came to visit him. So even before he came to live with me, I again started to look for my own apartment. The whole time he was living with me, it seemed the only two things he did were to sit in his room or go to his mother's. He didn't want to go out, or go to movies, but he did like to argue with the staff. I finally had more than I could take and I began to strike out at him.

In August of 1994, I had what I considered another milestone in my life. I got my first electric wheelchair. The "scooter", as it was called, helped me get around Baldwin on the run. Up until that time, people would often ask me, "Why don't you get a motor on your wheelchair?"

As the time for me to get my electric wheelchair/scooter got close, I looked forward to picking it out with great anticipation. A physical therapist gave me help in determining the right chair or scooter for me. One that would best fit my needs. After I got the scooter, I felt a great sense of freedom and independence. My days of being pushed, or rolling myself around Baldwin were over. Now, I was able to "drive" myself around town.

CHAPTER XIII
WHEELCHAIR ON THE TRACKS

They are slaves who fear to speak
for the fallen and the weak;
They are slaves who will not choose
hatred, scoffing, and abuse,
rather than in silence shrink
from the truth they needs must think;
They are slaves who dare not be
in the right with two or three.
———James Russell Lowell

In August of 1996, I found an apartment in downtown Baldwin. I lived by myself and went to the University of Wisconsin-Stout (UW-Stout). I was back to making my own breakfast, and doing my own laundry—and I loved it! I really enjoyed this time in my life.

While attending UW-Stout, I applied for and was given a job shredding paper at the university. As a result, I quit my shredding job at St. Croix Industries. Through the shredding job at the university, I was able to pay for a lot of my tuition.

Meanwhile, I was all over Baldwin on my electric scooter. I especially enjoyed Sundays, when I would drive over to visit some of my relatives. They had a big back yard that I would drive around in. It was a great place in which to turn "donuts". I drove a bit more carefully downtown, as I didn't want people talking, or the police to jail me for reckless driving.

At times, I would visit an uncle who lived in Baldwin and had a good garden. As I drove around the streets of Baldwin, I would sometimes pick up "road kill" and take it to my cousins house— NOT appreciated!

One time, as I was driving around Baldwin, I got the wheel of my scooter/chair stuck in the railroad tracks. I tried to go forward, I tried to go backward. I rocked the scooter from side to side. I tried to jump the chair up and down. I tried everything I could think of to free the wheel and get the chair off the tracks, but to no avail. I anxiously looked up and down the tracks—first one way, then the other. I breathed a sigh of relief that, at least for the moment, there was not a train coming.

Fortunately there were some people out for a walk. They saw my plight, and helped be off the tracks before something really serious happened. The feeling of being trapped on the railroad tracks is not unlike the feeling of being trapped in a body with a disability. You can struggle, fight, and strain until exhausted, but you cannot control whether or how you can move. It makes no difference how hard, or how desperately you try, or seek to wish away the obstacles, they are always there. The obstacles and barriers that keep you from easily functioning in everyday life never go away. But easy or difficult, function you must. At times, the especially difficult times, you need for someone walking by to stop, remove the barriers, and help you off the tracks.

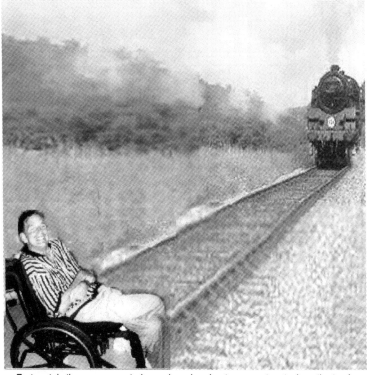

Fortunately there was no a train coming when I got my scooter stuck on the tracks.

67

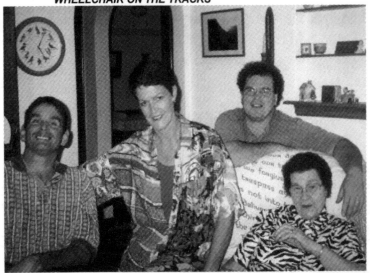

My sister, Betty, brother, Bob, and Mom

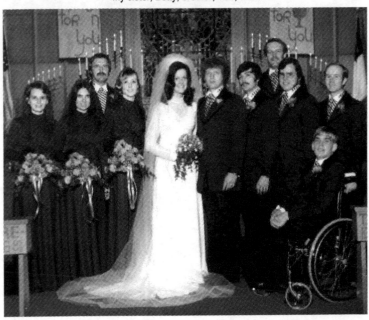

My sister, Betty's, wedding

CHAPTER XIV
MY BIGGEST MISTAKE

When you make a mistake, don't look back at
it long. Take the reason of the thing into your
mind and then look forward. Mistakes are
lessons of wisdom. The past cannot be
changed. The future is yet in your power.
——Hugh White

I think in everyone's life they make one mistake that will stick with them for the rest of their life. For me it came a year-and-a-half into my life at my apartment on Main Street, Baldwin.

My service provider began taking my attendants and moving them to other sites in order to help other people. One of the biggest challenges I've faced, is a dependable attendant service from my providers. Some attendants were good, some attendants were not good. One went to a group home where she could find a boyfriend. This left me in a position where I would sweep dirt from my floors into a pile and then wait for someone to come and pick it up. Sometimes it would be a long time before anyone would pick up the pile of dirt. I often thought of buying a house, but it was always too expensive.

In the fall of 1998, my service providers offered me

a chance to move into a house with two other people. I was told that I couldn't continue to live by myself because I was going down hill and was not taking care of myself. At first, I thought it was a good idea to move into the group house. It took until 1999 for them to find a house. It was a big, beautiful house.

I liked to go to movies and went almost every weekend. I knew the couple I would be living with, and I knew they didn't like to go anyplace. I was also told that they were mean. Still I went along with it, and after much delay, I finally moved into the house with them in the summer of 1999. My mother was living just a block away.

I went over to my mother's house a lot, especially on Sundays to watch the Green Bay Packers play football. In my childhood, about 1964, I was watching football and I became a Green Bay Packer fan. I've been an avid fan ever since. I remember watching the Packers play when it was fifteen degrees below zero. Being in the Wisconsin countryside, we had to turn the TV antenna toward La Crosse to pick up the signal. It was easy for me to be a Packer fan, but my mother's side of the family were all from Minnesota and are Viking fans—including my mom. There was a lot of good spirited disagreement and rivalry each Sunday afternoon. One Sunday, the Vikings were playing the Chicago

Bears. The Bears were to kick what would be the winning field goal. I cheered for them, and they missed!

I seem to recall reading somewhere that people who like the Vikings have a disability—However, I don't know if that is really true!

At this point in my life, school was very important to me. I did a lot of typing, which meant I almost lived in the computer lab at the university. At the same time, in connection with my advocacy work, I was on a statewide committee involved in a long-term redesign project of the social service system.

Going back to the subject of the house, it was a very nice, modern house. The service provider liked it a lot. After living there for awhile, I found out that the other two people were mentally ill. Looking back, I don't know if they wanted to live there or not. They just sat around the house, had arguments with the staff, and they did not want to do anything except watch T.V..

There are many reasons, that I feel the group home was a mistake: The staff, at times, would argue loudly among themselves; The residents argued about anything and everything— from the food not being right to problems with their money. At times I would turn my back so I wouldn't hear everybody arguing.

Perhaps this was one of the biggest reasons I feel that this group living situation was a mistake.

There were some positive things. It was in a nice location. It was only two blocks from the high school that I graduated from in 1979, and one block from my mom's house.

I started to go back to church again. I was raised in a small Baptist church in Hersey. When I moved to Baldwin, I attended Gethsemane Lutheran Church which was next door to the group home where I was living. I even joined the bell choir. Everyone was surprised. I made a lot of friendships at Gethsemane that have lasted many years.

Many of the staff at the group home were good people. When one of them got married, I was invited to the wedding. I had a good time. After the wedding ceremony, they invited me to go bar hopping . Some of the staff, at the home, also went to the University of Wisconsin-Stout. We would talk about our classes, go to sports events, or do other things together.

How often we wish for another chance to
make a fresh beginning,
A chance to blot our mistakes and change
failure into winning—
And it does not take a special time to make a
brand new start,
It only takes the deep desire to try with all
our heart
To live a little better, and to always be
forgiving
And to add a little "sunshine" to the
world in which we're living—
So never give up in despair and think
that you are through,
For there's always a tomorrow and a
chance to start anew.

——Helen Steiner Rice

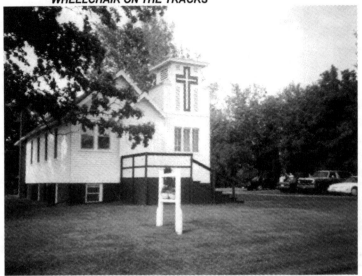

Hersey Church

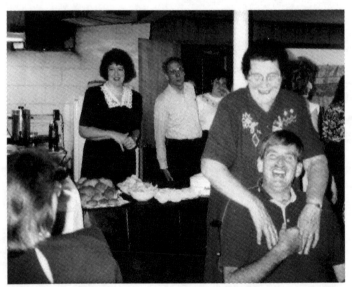

Fellowship dinner at Hersey Church.!

CHAPTER XV
NEW BEGINNINGS

The past is but the beginning of a begin-
ning and all that is and has been is but the
twilight of the dawn.
——*H. G. Wells*

As for the group home, there was still a lot of fighting
and arguing going on. In the summer of 2001, I began
looking for work again, and got a paper route. I used
my scooter to deliver the papers. I started experiencing
severe breathing problems and had to quit. I was sent to
Sacred Heart Hospital in Eau Claire for tests on my
breathing and swallowing. They recommended that a
baclofen pump be placed in my body. Baclofen is a
medicine to ease spasms that occur when muscles resist
being stretched. The pump would give me the medicine
continuously, and was to help with the problems I was
having swallowing and breathing. In October of 2001,
the baclofen pump was surgically placed in my abdo-
men.

December, 2001, I started working at the Baldwin
Memorial Hospital. I was a mail clerk and worked in
the mail room with the mail machine. My scooter took
me back and forth between home and my hospital jobs.

As for high school sports, you guessed it, I still went to the games. But now, rather than with the students, I went with teachers (Mr. Stein and Mr. Walker) that taught me when I was in high school.

The group home continued to get worse. Once, I was sick for four days, and no one would take me to the doctor. I became frustrated, insisting violently that something be done for me. They eventually had to lock me up in an institution.

In the end, I couldn't take living at the group home anymore. I did some things that were wrong, even hitting out at people. I got a new social worker, and in August, 2002, I moved out of the group home.

I moved into an apartment with another guy and another provider. He was older and had problems of his own, nevertheless, compared to the group home it was a good setup. Even so, it only lasted six months.

I started to go to movies and to my nephew's basketball games. I continued to go to work at the hospital on my scooter. In February of 2003, I had an accident. I was on my scooter when I was run over by a car. It was the other person's fault. After the accident, I was in the hospital for three days. They found that I had pneumonia and I was given a nebulizer.

In March, 2003, I had the privilege of going back to Madison to watch my nephew, Kyle, play in the high school state basketball tournament. Three months later, I was fighting for my life.

> *We know that we are expected to do our part, for Thou hast made us, not puppets, but persons with minds to think and wills to resolve. Make us willing to think, and think hard, clearly, and honestly, guided by Thy voice within us, and in accordance with the light Thou hast given us. May we never fail to do the best we can.*
>
> —From a prayer of Peter Marshall offered before the Senate of the United States, March 25, 1947

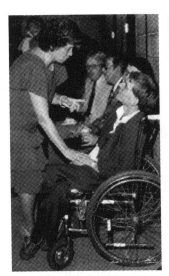 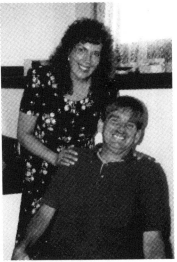

Phillip and Alice Swensson and their children; Gregg, Mary Alice, and Eric were special friends to our family. Here are a couple of pictures of me with:
Alice   —and with—   Mary Alice.

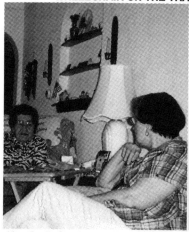 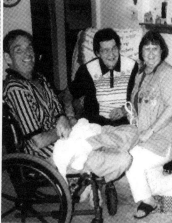

More family friends: Janice Walton   —and her daughter—   Diana Suderman

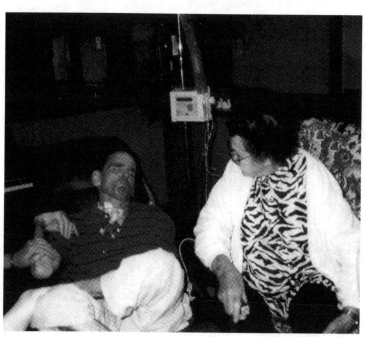

Lakeside Nursing Home

CHAPTER XVI
FIGHTING FOR MY LIFE

It is faith's work to claim and challenge lov-
ing-kindness out of all the roughest strokes of
God.

———Samuel Rutherford

Most of my adult life I've had days when I was so exhausted that I would sleep all day. In April of 2003,
something changed my life forever. I began having severe breathing problems and was again admitted to
Baldwin Memorial Hospital with pneumonia. I stayed
about a week, and then I was transferred to Sacred Heart
Hospital in Eau Claire.

The hospital staff began working on my swallowing. At first, I would hit out at them as they worked on
my baclofen pump. When I was strong enough to sit up
again, I recall many long days and nights sitting in my
room doing nothing. When I tired of that, I sat in the
hallway and just looked at people going by. I felt like a
picture on the wall, a piece of furniture, a face in the
crowd. No one stops to talk to the lone person lying in
bed, or the solitary person sitting in the hall. Unnoticed
and ignored, I sat with no place to go and nothing to do.

I'm sure you know the feeling. Maybe it has hap-

79

pened to you, and you hope it never happens again. The person with a disability doesn't need to wonder, they know it will happen again, and again and again.

The next time you visit a hospital, a nursing home, or any place where you see someone sitting alone, speak to them. *"A man finds joy in giving an apt reply-- and how good is a timely word!"* —Proverbs 15:23.

My pneumonia was getting bad. I was being given all kinds of breathing treatments.

Up until this time, I worked with different groups in Wisconsin on issues faced by those with disabilities. I remember the day when all this ended. It was while I was having some tests in the hospital, and I was told that during the swallowing test I aspirated. I was told, if I could no longer swallow, I would no longer be able to eat. I would have to go on a feeding tube.

I remember the day they put a feeding tube into me. I remember the last meal I ate.

The first time my mother came to see me, I was wearing a mask over my face. I remember my sister crying over me. They put me on a ventilator and I was on many I-Vs. I don't remember more, but when I woke up, a person from physical therapy was standing beside my bed with my brother, Bob, next to him. I couldn't talk. I couldn't tell Bob how much it meant for him to be there.

80

I had three long, terrible months in Sacred Heart Hospital. My dear sister, Betty, would come almost every day. They told me later that I almost died. It was then that I found out that the feeding tube meant, not only no more meat, but it also meant no more pizza, no more cookies, no more a lot of things..

Flowers and cards of every kind begin to arrive from all the people in Baldwin. The flowers and cards filled my hospital room. Someone said the town sold out of cards.

Because of the tracheotomy, I wasn't able to talk. They put me on a bed that would shake to help my breathing. I had so many different breathing treatments I couldn't count them. I was incapable of doing anything for myself. When I ended my stay at Sacred Heart, I was almost blind.

I had to totally depend on my caregivers, my family, my friends, and my God.

We do not need much time in order to love
God, to renew ourselves in His Presence,
to lift up our hearts towards Him,
to worship Him in the depths of our hearts,
to offer Him what we do and what we suffer.
——Fenelon

81

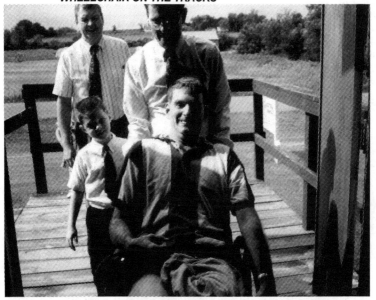

Pastor Jim Walton, his son, Dan (pushing me), and Dan's son, Mark.

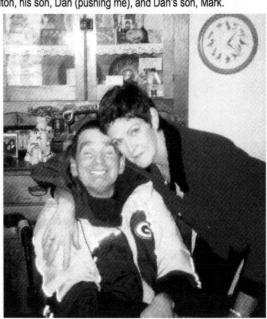

There's nothing quite
as nice as a hug from
your sister

82

CHAPTER XVII
LAKESIDE NURSING HOME

When obstacles and trials seem
Like prison-walls to be,
I do the little I can do,
And leave the rest to Thee.
—Frederick William Faber

In July of 2003, I went from Sacred Heart Hospital, in Eau Claire, to Lakeside nursing home in Chippewa Falls, Wisconsin. I was blind and could not talk. I used a word board to communicate.

I would sit in a long room near the piano and look out over an eating area. At times they would put a special vest on me to help my breathing. At other times, I would have to be suctioned to clear my breathing passages. Mother would drive from Baldwin to see me, and my sister would come from Eau Claire. I didn't know anyone at the home and had few visitors. They had a small staff at the home. I remember a nurse's aide, called Annett.

My eyesight began to come back. They worked a lot on trying to get me to swallow. The doctor said I would never eat again. I began to show my anger by hitting out at people.

83

Elisabeth Kübler-Ross in her book "On Death and Dying", Macmillan Publishing Company, 1969, gives 5 stages terminally ill persons may go through when they learn of their illness: Denial, Anger, Bargaining, Depression, Acceptance. They are sometimes called the "5 stages of Receiving Catastrophic News", or the "5 Stages of Grief". I don't know if I was going through these 5 stages one at a time, in some predefined order, or if anyone goes through them in order. I don't know if I was in denial, but I do know that this was a terribly dark period for me. Everything seemed meaningless and life was overwhelming. I wondered if there was any reason for me to go on, or even if I could go on.

> *There will come a time when you believe*
> *everything is finished. That will be the*
> *beginning.*
>
> ——*Louis L'Amour*

In August, I was able to go outside. The staff would take me for short walks in my wheelchair.

In the middle of September, I went back to my service provider.

CHAPTER XVIII
THE UNKNOWN FUTURE

My cloud of battle-dust may dim,
His veil of splendor curtain Him;
And, in the midnight of my fear,
I may not feel Him standing near:
But, as I lift mine eyes above,
His banner over me is love.
——Geranl Massey

I went back to the apartment in Baldwin. Soon, I got pneumonia and was admitted to the Baldwin hospital. The doctor who had worked with me before, worked on me again. I stayed in the Baldwin hospital for three months. They wanted me to go back to Eau Claire, but I didn't want to go. Then they wanted to send me back to Lakeside, but Lakeside didn't have enough staff. I still would not accept my not being able to eat. I revolted and got angry when a staff member from Lakeside came to see me. I ended up in a nursing home near Baldwin

I had another surgery to help me eat. It was unsuccessful. It was very difficult for me to accept that I could not eat. I was sent to another nursing home. Because I was unable to accept my inability to eat, I had a difficult time in these two nursing homes.

In addition, in one of the homes I didn't like the fact that I was put next door to a 90 year old man. I was young and resisted having to live where there were no young people. There were questionable conditions in one of the homes. I was depressed, I felt I was being ill-treated, and I did some terrible things of which I am not proud.

I want to grow to accept my disabilities. If anyone reading this book is fighting similar battles and having difficulty accepting what you cannot change, my desire for you, is what I desire for myself—it may have been best captured in the words of Reinhold Niebhur's familiar prayer:

> *God grant me*
> *Serenity to accept the things I cannot change,*
> *Courage to change the things that I can, and*
> *Wisdom to know the difference.*
> ——Reinhold Niebuhr

And my life goes on. With greater physical disabilities than when I started, but I am older and I hope wiser. As I said, I am still growing at accepting my disabilities—especially the ones I could once do, but now only miss. At times, I become angry at my circumstances, or at a society where, after almost a lifetime of advocating change, many of the barriers that hinder the ability of people with disabilities to easily function in everyday life still exist. Barriers that keep them from living independent and more productive lives. I feel driven, even now with my limitations, to be an advocate, a voice to speak for the people with disabilities.

I have often been told to let somebody else do this or that, somebody with fewer disabilities. "Roger, you can't do that." At other times, I have overheard someone say, "Roger is really sick, I'm afraid he won't recover this time." Each time I have surprised them. My sister, Betty, says my capacity for doing what others think impossible, or my ability to recover from severe illnesses, time and again is more than incredible good fortune. It is an unbelievable resilience.

I wonder if our purpose on earth is merely to sulk and languish in our misfortune? Are we to exhaust our strength only to better our own condition, or ease our pain alone? As long as I am able to wheel through life and cross the tracks, and as long as there are barriers that still need to be removed, I intend to do my part to make life better and easier for others with disabilities. Will you help me?

——ROGER RASMUSSEN

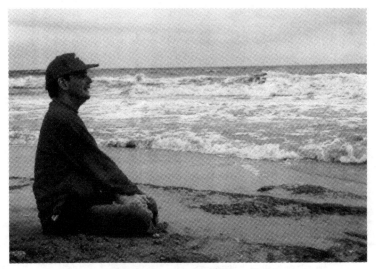

I know not what the future hath
Of marvel or surprise,
Assured alone that life and death
His mercy underlies.
————John Greenleaf Whittier

<u>APPENDICES</u>

APPENDIX A

TYPES OF CEREBRAL PALSY

There are four types of cerebral palsy. Each affects certain muscle groups and have certain disabilities associated with them:

Spastic Cerebral Palsy: Stiff and weak muscles.
Athetoid Cerebral Palsy: Uncontrolled and involuntary movements.
Ataxic Cerebral Palsy: Shaky movements and unsteady balance.
Mixed Cerebral Palsy: Combination of types, (usually Spastic and Athetoid).

Although Cerebral Palsy is not curable, there are many cerebral palsy treatment options available to help a child with cerebral palsy lead a more productive and independent life. Cerebral palsy does not go away when the person becomes an adult. Many individuals struggle to transition into adulthood.

> *It is not a question of patronizing philanthropy towards disabled people. They do not need the patronage of the non-disabled. It is not for them to adapt to the dominant and dominating world of the so-called non-disabled. It is for us to adapt our understanding of a common humanity; to learn of the richness of how human life is diverse; to recognize the presence of disability in our human midst as an enrichment of our diversity.*
> ——Nelson Mandela

90

APPENDIX B

When Meeting, Writing or Speaking About a Person With a Disability

Information supplied by
Courage Center, Minneapolis, Minn.
www.courage.org

When Meeting
a Person with a Disability.

Be yourself. Treat me as you would anyone else you meet.

Respect my right to let you know what kind of help I need. Use good judgment on whether or not to ask if I need your assistance.

Talk directly to me not to the person who might be with me. And, if I'm in a wheelchair, try to put yourself at my eye level.

If I have a speech disorder, I may be hard to understand. So, ask me to repeat what I say until you understand or ask another person to help.

If I'm deaf and no interpreter is present, talk to me using a normal tone and rhythm of speech. If you speak rapidly you may need to slow down somewhat. Consider using a notepad and pencil.

When my service dog is in a harness, don't pet him. He's working and cannot play.

Be considerate and patient with the extra time I might need to do or say things.

Never start to push my wheelchair without asking if you may do so. Let me tell you how to push my chair over inaccessible curbs or stairs.

If I have a visual impairment, ask if you can help. If needed, let me take your arm for guidance.

Remember that I have many interests other than those associated with my disability. I'm a person like anyone else; I just happen to have a disability.

When Writing or Speaking
About a Person with a Disability.

Always put the person first, then the disability. Say or write "person with a disability" rather than disabled person.

Disability is defined as a functional limitation that interferes with a person's ability to walk, hear, see, talk and learn.

Barriers are what "handicap" a person's ability to easily function in everyday life—not a person's disability.

Don't be concerned if you find yourself using words like "see" to a person who is blind or "hear" to a person who is deaf. These words won't offend.

Do not refer to a person in a wheelchair as "confined" to a wheelchair. It's better to say or write "uses a wheelchair."

Do not say "normal person" as compared to a person with a disability. Say able-bodied or non-disabled. Better yet, say nothing at all.

Avoid such words as victim, stricken with, crippled, mute, deaf and dumb or afflicted. For example, refer to a person who has had a stroke as a stroke survivor not as a stroke victim.

Do not say arthritic or cerebral palsied. It's better to say, "he has arthritis" or "she has cerebral palsy."

Do not say birth defect. It's better to say, a person who has had a disability since birth or that she has a congenital disability.

Remember that a person with a disability is a person like anyone else, they just happen to have a disability

WHEELCHAIR ON THE TRACKS